MIRACLE CBD

Unlock the Healing Power of Cannabidiol for Inflammation and Chronic Pain Relief

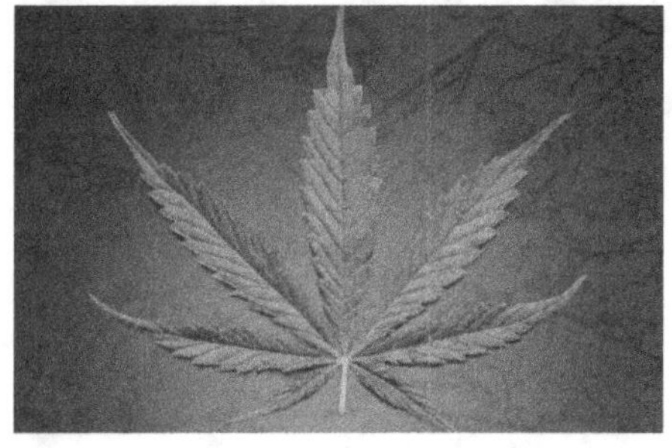

Katherine Peters

Table of Contents

Introduction

The CBD Revolution - Nature's Answer to Chronic Pain

Kate Wilson had always been an active person. At 42, she was a devoted mother of two, a successful marketing executive, and an avid runner who had completed three marathons. But all that changed one fateful morning when she woke up with an excruciating pain in her lower back. What she initially dismissed as a temporary discomfort soon became a relentless, debilitating condition that would alter the course of her life.

For the next two years, Kate's world shrank. The pain was constant, radiating from her lower back down to her legs. Simple tasks like getting out of bed or picking up her children became monumental challenges. She cycled through a carousel of treatments - physical therapy, chiropractic care, acupuncture, and finally, powerful prescription painkillers. While the opioids provided some relief, they left her feeling foggy and disconnected from her life. Kate found herself spiraling into depression, watching her career stall and her relationships strain under the weight of her condition.

It was during one of her lowest moments, contemplating whether she'd ever regain any semblance of her former life, that Kate stumbled upon an article about CBD. Desperate for an alternative, she decided to give it a try. Starting with a low dose of CBD oil, Kate was cautiously optimistic. Within weeks, she noticed a subtle shift - the edge of her pain seemed to dull, and her sleep improved. Encouraged, she worked with a CBD-friendly doctor to optimize her dosage and delivery method.

Six months into her CBD regimen, Kate's transformation was nothing short of remarkable. Her pain levels had decreased dramatically, allowing her to reduce her opioid use significantly. She was sleeping better, her mood had improved, and she had started to regain her physical strength. A year later, Kate completed a 5K run - a feat that would have been unimaginable just months earlier. While she wasn't entirely pain-free, CBD had given Kate her life back, allowing her to be present for her family and reengage with her career.

Kate's story is not unique. Across the globe, countless individuals are discovering the potential of CBD to manage chronic pain and reclaim their lives. Her journey from despair to hope mirrors the broader narrative of CBD's emergence as a promising solution in the face of a global chronic pain crisis.

The Global Impact of Chronic Pain

Chronic pain is a silent epidemic that affects millions worldwide, transcending age, gender, and socioeconomic boundaries. According to the World Health Organization, approximately 1.5 billion people globally suffer from chronic pain. In the United States alone, it's estimated that over 50 million adults experience chronic pain, with nearly 20 million enduring high-impact chronic pain that significantly limits life or work activities.

The ramifications of this epidemic extend far beyond individual suffering. Chronic pain exacts a tremendous toll on global economies, healthcare systems, and societal well-being. In the U.S., the annual cost of chronic pain is estimated to be $635 billion, surpassing the yearly costs for cancer, heart disease, and diabetes combined. This figure includes direct medical costs, lost productivity, and disability programs.

Moreover, the emotional and psychological impact of chronic pain cannot be overstated. Those living with persistent pain often experience depression, anxiety, and sleep disorders. Relationships suffer, careers are derailed, and the overall quality of life diminishes significantly. The opioid crisis, largely fueled by attempts to manage chronic pain, has added another layer of complexity and urgency to this issue.

Traditional pain management strategies, while beneficial for many, come with their own set of challenges. Non-steroidal anti-inflammatory drugs (NSAIDs) can lead to gastrointestinal issues and increased cardiovascular risks with long-term use. Opioids, while effective for severe pain, carry the risks of addiction, tolerance, and a host of side effects. Surgery and interventional procedures are invasive and don't always provide long-term relief.

It's within this context that the need for alternative, effective, and safer pain management solutions has become increasingly urgent. Enter CBD - a compound that has sparked a revolution in how we approach chronic pain and inflammation.

The Emergence of CBD: A Brief History

Cannabidiol, or CBD, is one of over 100 cannabinoids found in the Cannabis sativa plant. Unlike its more famous cousin, tetrahydrocannabinol (THC), CBD doesn't produce a "high" or psychoactive effect. This crucial difference has allowed CBD to navigate legal and social barriers more easily, paving the way for its exploration as a therapeutic agent.

The history of CBD dates back to 1940 when it was first isolated from the cannabis plant by American chemist Roger Adams. However, its structure wasn't fully elucidated until 1963 by Israeli scientist Raphael Mechoulam, often referred to as the "father of cannabis research."

Despite these early discoveries, CBD remained largely overlooked for decades, overshadowed by the controversy surrounding THC and marijuana use. It wasn't until the late 1990s and early 2000s that interest in CBD began to resurge, driven by a growing body of preclinical research suggesting its potential therapeutic properties.

A pivotal moment in CBD's journey to the mainstream came in 2013 with the story of Charlotte Figi, a young girl with a severe form of epilepsy. After finding significant relief using a CBD-rich cannabis extract, Charlotte's story captured national attention, sparking a renewed interest in CBD's potential medical applications.

Since then, research into CBD has exploded. Studies have explored its effects on various conditions, including chronic pain, anxiety, epilepsy, and inflammation. In 2018, the FDA approved Epidiolex, a CBD-based medication for certain forms of epilepsy, marking the first federal approval of a cannabis-derived drug.

Concurrently, changes in cannabis legislation across many countries and states have made CBD more accessible. The 2018 Farm Bill in the United States legalized hemp-derived CBD at the federal level, opening the floodgates for CBD products in the marketplace.

Today, CBD stands at the forefront of a new paradigm in pain management and overall wellness. Its potential to provide relief without the side effects associated with many traditional pain medications has captured the attention of both the medical community and the public at large.

As we examine deeper into the world of CBD throughout this book, we'll explore the science behind its effects, its potential applications for various pain conditions, and how it might be integrated into a comprehensive pain management strategy. From Kate's story to the broader global context, it's clear that CBD represents more than just another treatment option - it embodies hope for millions suffering from chronic pain, offering the promise of reclaiming lives once thought lost to persistent suffering.

The CBD revolution is not just about a single compound; it's about reimagining our approach to pain and wellness. As we stand on the cusp of this new era in pain management, the potential of CBD to transform lives, like Kate's, offers a compelling reason to explore this natural, powerful alternative.

Chapter 1

Demystifying CBD - The Healing Compound

In recent years, CBD has emerged from relative obscurity to become a household name, touted for its potential therapeutic benefits. Yet, despite its growing popularity, there remains a cloud of mystery and misconception surrounding this compound. In this chapter, we'll peel back the layers of complexity to reveal the true nature of CBD, its origins, and how it interacts with our bodies. By understanding the fundamentals, we can better appreciate the potential of this remarkable substance.

The Origins of CBD in the Cannabis Plant

To truly understand CBD, we must first explore its source: the Cannabis sativa plant. Cannabis has been cultivated by humans for thousands of years, with its use dating back to ancient civilizations in China, India, and the Middle East. The plant has been used for a variety of purposes, including fiber production, religious ceremonies, and medicinal applications.

Cannabis sativa is a complex plant containing over 400 chemical entities, of which more than 100 are cannabinoids. Cannabinoids are compounds unique to the cannabis plant, and CBD is one of the most abundant among them.

Within the cannabis plant, cannabinoids are primarily found in the resin produced by the plant's trichomes. Trichomes are tiny, hair-like structures that cover the surface of the plant, particularly concentrated on the flowers (or buds) of female plants. These trichomes serve as the plant's natural defense mechanism, protecting it from pests and environmental stressors.

It's important to note that while CBD can be found in all varieties of cannabis, it's typically most abundant in hemp - a variety of Cannabis sativa that contains very low levels of THC (less than 0.3% by dry weight). This distinction is crucial, as it allows for the legal cultivation and use of hemp-derived CBD in many jurisdictions where marijuana (cannabis with higher THC content) remains restricted.

The CBD Extraction Process

Extracting CBD from the cannabis plant is a sophisticated process that requires careful attention to detail to ensure purity and potency. There are several methods used for CBD extraction, each with its own advantages and drawbacks. Let's explore some of the most common techniques:

1. **CO2 Extraction**: This is considered the gold standard in the industry due to its ability to produce pure, high-quality CBD without the use of toxic solvents. In this method, carbon dioxide is pressurized into a supercritical fluid, which then acts as a solvent to extract the CBD from the plant material. The CO2 is then allowed to evaporate, leaving behind pure CBD oil. While this method is extremely effective, it requires expensive equipment and expertise to execute properly.

2. **Ethanol Extraction**: This method involves soaking the plant material in high-grade grain alcohol to extract the cannabinoids. The alcohol is then evaporated to leave behind the CBD oil. This method is efficient and can be done at large scales, but it may also extract unwanted compounds like chlorophyll, which can affect the taste and color of the final product.

3. **Oil Extraction**: This is one of the oldest methods of extraction and involves heating the plant material in a

carrier oil (like olive oil) to extract the cannabinoids. While this method is simple and inexpensive, it's less efficient than other methods and produces lower concentrations of CBD.

4. **Hydrocarbon Extraction**: This method uses solvents like butane or propane to extract CBD. While it can be effective, it's potentially dangerous due to the flammable nature of these solvents and may leave behind toxic residues if not done properly.

After extraction, the resulting CBD oil often undergoes further refinement processes to remove any remaining plant materials or unwanted compounds. The final product can range from full-spectrum CBD oil (containing all the plant's cannabinoids and terpenes) to CBD isolate (pure CBD with all other compounds removed).

Understanding the Endocannabinoid System

To comprehend how CBD works in the body, we need to explore one of the most fascinating biological systems you've probably never heard of: the endocannabinoid system (ECS). Discovered in the early 1990s, the ECS is a complex cell-signaling system that plays a crucial role in regulating a wide range of bodily functions.

Think of the ECS as your body's internal balancing act. Just as a tightrope walker constantly makes tiny adjustments to maintain balance, the ECS works tirelessly to keep your body in a state of homeostasis - a condition of optimal functioning where everything is just right.

The ECS is composed of three main elements:

1. **Endocannabinoids**: These are molecules produced naturally by your body. They're similar to the cannabinoids found in the cannabis plant, hence the name "endo-cannabinoids" (endo meaning "within"). The two key endocannabinoids identified so far are anandamide (AEA) and 2-arachidonoylglycerol (2-AG).

2. **Cannabinoid Receptors**: These are found throughout your body and act as landing sites for both endocannabinoids and plant-derived cannabinoids like CBD. The two main types are CB1 receptors (primarily in the central nervous system) and CB2 receptors (mainly in the peripheral nervous system, especially immune cells).

3. **Enzymes**: These are responsible for breaking down endocannabinoids once they've carried out their function.

To better understand how this system works, let's use an analogy:

Imagine your body as a bustling city. The endocannabinoids are like the city's maintenance crew, constantly patrolling the streets (your body) looking for problems to fix. The cannabinoid receptors are like the crew's communication devices, alerting them to issues that need attention. When the maintenance crew (endocannabinoids) receives an alert through their devices (receptors), they rush to the scene to restore order. Once the job is done, the enzymes act like the cleanup crew, clearing away the endocannabinoids to prevent overaccumulation.

This system helps regulate numerous functions, including:

- Pain sensation

- Mood

- Appetite

- Sleep

- Memory

- Immune function

- Reproductive system function

- Stress response

The discovery of the ECS has revolutionized our understanding of health and disease, providing new targets for therapeutic interventions. It's within this context that CBD's potential becomes truly exciting.

CBD and the Endocannabinoid System

Unlike THC, which binds directly to cannabinoid receptors, CBD's interaction with the ECS is more nuanced. Rather than binding directly to the receptors, CBD appears to work indirectly, influencing the ECS in several ways:

1. **Inhibiting Enzyme Action**: CBD can inhibit the enzymes that break down endocannabinoids, potentially prolonging their effects.

2. **Increasing Endocannabinoid Production**: Some research suggests CBD might enhance the body's production of endocannabinoids.

3. **Binding to Other Receptors**: CBD can interact with other receptors in the body, such as serotonin receptors, which may contribute to its effects on mood and pain perception.

These interactions help explain why CBD might have such a wide range of potential therapeutic applications, from pain relief to anxiety reduction.

CBD vs. THC: Clearing the Confusion

While CBD and THC are both cannabinoids found in the cannabis plant, they have distinct properties and effects. Understanding these differences is crucial for appreciating CBD's therapeutic potential without the stigma often associated with cannabis use.

Chemical Structure:

CBD and THC have the exact same molecular formula: 21 carbon atoms, 30 hydrogen atoms, and 2 oxygen atoms. However, a slight difference in how these atoms are arranged accounts for the dramatically different effects of the two compounds.

Psychoactive Effects:

The most well-known difference between CBD and THC is their effect on cognition and perception. THC is responsible for the "high" associated with marijuana use. It binds directly to CB1 receptors in the brain, altering perception, mood, and consciousness. CBD, on the other hand, does not produce a high. It doesn't bind directly to CB1 receptors and can even mitigate some of THC's psychoactive effects.

Medical Applications:

Both CBD and THC have potential therapeutic applications, but they're often used for different purposes:

- THC is commonly used for conditions like chronic pain, muscle spasticity, glaucoma, insomnia, and low appetite.

- CBD is being studied for its potential in treating anxiety, depression, seizures, inflammation, and chronic pain, among other conditions.

Side Effects:

THC can cause side effects such as increased heart rate, coordination problems, dry mouth, red eyes, slower reaction times, and memory loss. It can also induce anxiety or paranoia in some users.

CBD is generally well-tolerated, with side effects, when they occur, typically being mild. These can include fatigue, changes in appetite, and diarrhea. Importantly, CBD doesn't impair cognitive function or motor skills.

Legal Status:

The legal status of CBD and THC varies widely depending on jurisdiction. In many places, THC remains a controlled substance due to its psychoactive properties. CBD derived from hemp (cannabis with less than 0.3% THC) was made federally legal in the United States with the 2018 Farm Bill, though regulations can vary at the state level.

Drug Testing:

Standard drug tests look for THC or its metabolites and do not detect CBD. However, some CBD products may contain trace amounts of THC, which could potentially result in a positive drug test in rare cases.

Addressing Common Misconceptions

As CBD has gained popularity, several misconceptions have arisen. Let's address some of the most common:

Misconception 1: CBD gets you high.

Reality: CBD is non-intoxicating and does not produce a high. Any psychoactive effects from a "CBD product" are likely due to THC content.

Misconception 2: CBD is sedating.

Reality: While some people report feeling relaxed with CBD, research suggests it may actually be alerting in low to moderate doses. Higher doses may have a more sedative effect.

Misconception 3: CBD works immediately.

Reality: While some people may feel effects quickly, especially with methods like vaping, for many conditions, it may take consistent use over weeks or even months to see significant benefits.

Misconception 4: More CBD is always better.

Reality: CBD often works best at moderate doses. In some cases, lower doses may be more effective than higher ones, a phenomenon known as the biphasic effect.

Misconception 5: CBD cures everything.

Reality: While CBD shows promise for many conditions, it's not a panacea. More research is needed to fully understand its effects and optimal use for various health issues.

Misconception 6: All CBD products are the same.

Reality: The quality, purity, and potency of CBD products can vary widely. It's crucial to choose products from reputable manufacturers who provide third-party lab testing results.

Misconception 7: CBD is completely risk-free.

Reality: While CBD is generally well-tolerated, it can interact with certain medications and may cause side effects in some people. It's always best to consult with a healthcare provider before starting CBD, especially if you're on other medications.

Chapter 2

The Science of Inflammation and Pain

Pain is an universal human experience, yet it remains one of the most complex and challenging aspects of medicine. To truly understand the potential of CBD in pain management, we must first examine the intricate world of pain and inflammation. This chapter will explore the prevalence of chronic pain, unravel the biological processes behind inflammation, and examine the current approaches to pain management along with their limitations.

The Epidemic of Chronic Pain

Chronic pain is not just a medical issue; it's a societal crisis that affects millions of lives worldwide. The numbers are staggering and paint a picture of a silent epidemic that touches every corner of our global community.

Global Prevalence:

According to the Global Burden of Disease Study, chronic pain affects approximately 1.5 billion people worldwide.

This means that roughly 20% of the global population is living with some form of persistent pain. The prevalence varies by region and specific condition, but the overall impact is undeniable.

In the United States alone, the situation is equally alarming:

- The Centers for Disease Control and Prevention (CDC) estimates that 50 million American adults (about 20.4% of the adult population) suffer from chronic pain.

- Of these, 19.6 million (8% of adults) experience high-impact chronic pain, which frequently limits life or work activities.

- Chronic pain is more prevalent among women (21.7%) compared to men (19.0%).

- The prevalence increases with age, with 30.8% of adults aged 65 and older reporting chronic pain.

Economic Impact:

The financial burden of chronic pain is enormous, affecting individuals, healthcare systems, and national economies:

- In the United States, the annual cost of chronic pain is estimated to be between $560-635 billion. This includes direct medical costs, lost productivity, and disability programs.

- Chronic pain is the leading cause of long-term disability in the United States, affecting more Americans than diabetes, heart disease, and cancer combined.

- Globally, lower back pain alone is estimated to cost the global economy $585 billion annually in medical expenses and lost productivity.

Societal and Personal Impact:

Beyond the numbers, chronic pain has a profound impact on individuals and society:

- **Mental Health**: Chronic pain is closely linked with mental health issues. Up to 85% of patients with chronic pain are affected by severe depression.

- **Quality of Life**: Persistent pain can significantly reduce quality of life, affecting sleep, cognitive function, relationships, and overall well-being.

- **Opioid Crisis**: The attempt to manage chronic pain has contributed to the opioid epidemic, with an estimated 128 people in the United States dying every day from opioid overdoses.

- **Workforce Impact**: Chronic pain is a leading cause of work absenteeism and reduced productivity, with an estimated 323 million workdays lost annually in the U.S. alone.

These statistics underscore the urgent need for effective, safe, and accessible pain management solutions. As we explore the potential of CBD, it's crucial to keep in mind the vast number of lives that could be improved by advancements in this field.

Understanding Inflammation: The Body's Double-Edged Sword

Inflammation is a fundamental biological process that plays a crucial role in our body's defense mechanisms. It's our immune system's response to harmful stimuli, such as pathogens, damaged cells, or irritants. However, like many biological processes, inflammation can be both beneficial and detrimental, depending on its duration and context.

Acute Inflammation: The Body's First Line of Defense

Acute inflammation is a short-term response that typically lasts for hours to days. It's a vital part of the healing process and is characterized by five cardinal signs:

1. Redness (Rubor): Caused by increased blood flow to the affected area.

2. Heat (Calor): Also due to increased blood flow and metabolic activity.

3. Swelling (Tumor): Results from fluid accumulation in tissues.

4. Pain (Dolor): Caused by the release of chemicals that stimulate nerve endings.

5. Loss of Function (Functio laesa): Due to the combination of pain, swelling, and potential tissue damage.

The Process of Acute Inflammation:

1. **Recognition**: Specialized cells in the immune system recognize a threat.

2. **Recruitment**: These cells release chemical signals (cytokines and chemokines) that attract more immune cells to the site.

3. **Elimination**: Immune cells work to neutralize or eliminate the threat.

4. **Resolution**: Once the threat is dealt with, anti-inflammatory processes begin to restore tissue to its normal state.

Acute inflammation is generally beneficial, helping the body fight off infections and heal injuries. However, problems arise when inflammation becomes chronic.

Chronic Inflammation: When the Body's Defense Turns Against Itself

Chronic inflammation occurs when the inflammatory response persists for months or even years. This can happen due to:

- Failure to eliminate the initial cause of inflammation

- Exposure to a low level of a particular irritant over a long period

- An autoimmune disorder where the immune system attacks healthy tissue

- Recurrent episodes of acute inflammation

Unlike acute inflammation, chronic inflammation often doesn't have obvious external signs. It's a smoldering process that can damage tissues over time, contributing to a variety of health problems, including:

- Cardiovascular diseases

- Type 2 diabetes

- Cancer

- Neurodegenerative diseases like Alzheimer's and Parkinson's

- Rheumatoid arthritis

- Chronic pain conditions

The Inflammation-Pain Connection:

Inflammation and pain are closely intertwined. While acute inflammation can cause temporary pain as part of the healing process, chronic inflammation can lead to persistent pain. This happens through several mechanisms:

1. **Sensitization**: Inflammatory mediators can make pain receptors (nociceptors) more sensitive, lowering the threshold for pain signals.

2. **Tissue Damage**: Ongoing inflammation can cause tissue damage, leading to more pain.

3. **Central Sensitization**: Prolonged pain signals can cause changes in the central nervous system, making it more responsive to pain inputs.

Understanding this connection is crucial for developing effective pain management strategies, including the potential use of anti-inflammatory compounds like CBD.

The management of chronic pain has long been a challenge in medicine. Current approaches often involve a combination of pharmacological and non-pharmacological interventions. While these methods can be effective for many patients, they each come with their own set of limitations and potential risks.

1. Non-Steroidal Anti-Inflammatory Drugs (NSAIDs)

NSAIDs like ibuprofen and naproxen are commonly used for pain relief and to reduce inflammation.

Benefits:

- Effective for mild to moderate pain

- Available over-the-counter

- Can reduce inflammation

Drawbacks and Risks:

- Gastrointestinal issues, including ulcers and bleeding

- Increased risk of heart attack and stroke with long-term use

- Kidney damage with prolonged use

- Not suitable for all patients, especially those with certain health conditions

2. Opioids

Opioids are powerful pain relievers that work by binding to opioid receptors in the brain and body.

Benefits:

- Highly effective for severe pain

- Can provide significant relief for patients with advanced diseases

Drawbacks and Risks:

- High risk of addiction and dependence

- Tolerance development, requiring increasing doses over time

- Respiratory depression, which can be life-threatening

- Constipation and other side effects

- Contributes to the ongoing opioid crisis

3. Acetaminophen (Paracetamol)

Acetaminophen is a pain reliever that works differently from NSAIDs and doesn't reduce inflammation.

Benefits:

- Effective for mild to moderate pain

- Generally well-tolerated

- Doesn't cause gastrointestinal issues like NSAIDs

Drawbacks and Risks:

- Can cause severe liver damage if taken in high doses or combined with alcohol

- Not effective for inflammatory conditions

- May not be sufficient for severe pain

4. Corticosteroids

Corticosteroids are powerful anti-inflammatory drugs used for various conditions.

Benefits:

- Highly effective at reducing inflammation

- Can provide significant pain relief in inflammatory conditions

Drawbacks and Risks:

- Long-term use can lead to serious side effects, including osteoporosis, weight gain, and increased risk of infections

- Can cause adrenal suppression

- Not suitable for long-term use in many cases

5. Antidepressants and Anticonvulsants

Certain antidepressants and anticonvulsants are used off-label for chronic pain, especially neuropathic pain.

Benefits:

- Can be effective for certain types of pain, particularly neuropathic pain

- May help with associated conditions like depression and anxiety

Drawbacks and Risks:

- Can have significant side effects, including drowsiness, weight gain, and sexual dysfunction

- May take weeks to become effective

- Not all patients respond to these medications

6. Physical Therapy and Exercise

Non-pharmacological approaches like physical therapy and exercise are often recommended for chronic pain management.

Benefits:

- Can improve function and quality of life

- No risk of drug-related side effects

- May provide long-term benefits

Drawbacks and Limitations:

- May not provide immediate pain relief

- Requires consistent effort and time commitment from patients

- May not be sufficient as a standalone treatment for severe pain

7. Psychological Interventions

Cognitive-behavioral therapy and other psychological approaches are increasingly recognized as important in pain management.

Benefits:

- Can help patients develop coping strategies

- May reduce reliance on medications

- Addresses the psychological impact of chronic pain

Drawbacks and Limitations:

- May not directly address the physical causes of pain

- Requires patient engagement and commitment

- Access to qualified therapists may be limited in some areas

8. Interventional Procedures

These include injections, nerve blocks, and more invasive procedures like spinal cord stimulation.

Benefits:

- Can provide significant relief for specific types of pain

- May reduce reliance on oral medications

Drawbacks and Risks:

- Invasive procedures carry risks of complications

- Effects may be temporary, requiring repeated procedures

- Not suitable for all types of pain or all patients

While these conventional approaches to pain management have their place and can be effective for many patients, they all have limitations:

1. **Incomplete Relief**: Many patients do not achieve complete pain relief with current treatments.

2. **Side Effects**: Most pharmacological treatments come with the risk of side effects, some of which can be severe.

3. **Tolerance and Dependence**: Some pain medications, particularly opioids, can lead to tolerance and dependence.

4. **Lack of Long-Term Solutions**: Many treatments address symptoms without targeting the underlying causes of chronic pain.

5. **Individual Variability**: Pain is a subjective experience, and treatments that work for one person may not work for another.

6. **Multifaceted Nature of Pain**: Chronic pain often involves complex interactions between physical, psychological, and social factors, which are not all addressed by conventional treatments.

7. **Cost and Access**: Some treatments, particularly newer or more specialized ones, may be expensive or not readily accessible to all patients.

These limitations highlight the need for new approaches to pain management that can provide effective relief with fewer side effects and risks. This is where alternative treatments like CBD enter the picture, offering potential new avenues for managing chronic pain and inflammation.

As we move forward in this book, we'll explore how CBD interacts with the body's pain and inflammation pathways, potentially offering a new tool in the fight against chronic pain. By understanding the complexities of pain and inflammation, as well as the limitations of current treatments, we can better appreciate the potential role of CBD in comprehensive pain management strategies.

The exploration of CBD and other cannabinoids represents an exciting frontier in pain research. While it's not a panacea, CBD offers hope for many suffering from chronic pain, potentially providing a new option with a different risk-benefit profile compared to conventional treatments. As we journey deeper into the science of CBD in the following chapters, we'll examine how it might address some of the limitations of current pain management approaches, offering new possibilities for those living with chronic pain.

Chapter 3

CBD's Mechanism of Action

As we go deeper into the world of CBD and its potential for pain management, it's crucial to understand how this remarkable compound interacts with our bodies at a molecular level. In this chapter, we'll explore the intricate mechanisms through which CBD exerts its effects, focusing on its interactions with various receptors, its role in pain modulation, and its anti-inflammatory properties. By understanding these processes, we can better appreciate the potential of CBD as a therapeutic agent and its place in the broader landscape of pain management.

CBD's Interactions with Bodily Receptors

Unlike many pharmaceutical drugs that typically target a single receptor or pathway, CBD's effects are multifaceted, interacting with numerous receptors and systems throughout the body. This complex interplay contributes to CBD's wide range of potential therapeutic effects. Let's examine some of the key receptors and systems with which CBD interacts:

1. **Endocannabinoid System (ECS) Receptors**

While CBD doesn't bind directly to the main cannabinoid receptors (CB1 and CB2) in the same way that THC does, it still influences the endocannabinoid system in several important ways:

a) **CB1 Receptors**: These are primarily found in the central nervous system. While CBD doesn't activate CB1 receptors directly, it can act as a negative allosteric modulator. This means it can change the receptor's shape, making it harder for other cannabinoids (like THC) to bind to it. This is part of the reason why CBD can mitigate some of the psychoactive effects of THC.

b) **CB2 Receptors**: These are mainly found in the peripheral nervous system, especially in immune cells. CBD has been shown to have a complex relationship with CB2 receptors, sometimes appearing to block them and other times activating them indirectly.

c) **Endocannabinoid Levels**: CBD can increase levels of endocannabinoids like anandamide by inhibiting the enzymes that break them down. This allows these natural cannabinoids to have a more prolonged effect in the body.

2. Serotonin Receptors

CBD interacts with several serotonin receptors, most notably the 5-HT1A receptor. This interaction is thought to be behind some of CBD's anxiolytic (anti-anxiety) and antidepressant-like effects. The 5-HT1A receptor is involved in a wide array of processes, including pain perception, nausea, sleep, appetite, and anxiety.

3. Vanilloid Receptors

CBD is a potent activator of the TRPV1 receptor, also known as the vanilloid receptor 1. This receptor is involved in pain perception, inflammation, and body temperature regulation. By activating TRPV1, CBD may help desensitize pain pathways over time.

4. GPR55 Receptor

CBD has been shown to block the GPR55 receptor, which is sometimes called the "third cannabinoid receptor." This receptor is involved in regulating blood pressure and bone density, and its overactivation has been linked to osteoporosis and certain types of cancer.

5. **PPARγ Receptor**

CBD can activate the PPARγ (peroxisome proliferator-activated receptor gamma) nuclear receptor. This interaction is thought to be behind some of CBD's potential anti-inflammatory and neuroprotective effects.

6. **Adenosine Receptors**

CBD may enhance signaling of the A2A adenosine receptor. This could explain some of its anti-inflammatory and pain-relieving effects, as activation of A2A receptors has been shown to reduce inflammation and pain.

Understanding Pain Modulation and CBD's Influence

To appreciate how CBD might influence pain perception, it's essential to understand the concept of pain modulation. Pain is not simply a one-way signal from an injured body part to the brain. Instead, it's a complex process that can be amplified or diminished at various points along the pain pathway.

The Pain Pathway:

1. **Nociception**: This is the process by which potentially harmful stimuli (like heat, pressure, or chemical irritants) are detected by specialized nerve endings called nociceptors.

2. **Transmission**: The pain signal is transmitted through nerve fibers to the spinal cord.

3. **Spinal Cord Processing**: In the dorsal horn of the spinal cord, the pain signal can be modulated (enhanced or inhibited) before being sent to the brain.

4. **Perception**: The brain processes the pain signal, leading to the conscious experience of pain.

Pain Modulation:

Pain modulation occurs at various levels of this pathway, particularly in the spinal cord and brain. The body has built-in pain modulation systems, including:

1. Descending Pain Inhibitory Pathways: These are neural pathways that can dampen pain signals. They're activated by the brain and can release neurotransmitters like endorphins, serotonin, and norepinephrine to reduce pain perception.

2. Gate Control Theory: This theory proposes that non-painful input can close the "gates" to painful input, inhibiting pain sensation from traveling to the central nervous system.

CBD's Influence on Pain Modulation:

CBD appears to influence pain modulation through several mechanisms:

1. **Enhancing Endocannabinoid Signaling**: By increasing levels of endocannabinoids like anandamide, CBD may enhance the body's natural pain-modulating capabilities. Endocannabinoids are involved in regulating pain sensation, and higher levels could lead to reduced pain perception.

2. **Activating Serotonin Receptors**: CBD's interaction with 5-HT1A receptors may contribute to pain modulation. Serotonin is involved in descending pain inhibitory pathways, and by enhancing serotonin signaling, CBD could help dampen pain signals.

3. **Desensitizing TRPV1 Receptors**: While initial activation of TRPV1 receptors by CBD might cause a perception of pain, over time, this activation can lead to desensitization of the pain pathway, potentially resulting in an analgesic effect.

4. **Reducing Inflammation**: By decreasing inflammation (through mechanisms we'll explore later), CBD may indirectly reduce pain by addressing one of its root causes.

5. **Anxiolytic Effects**: Pain perception can be amplified by anxiety and stress. By reducing anxiety, CBD may indirectly help in pain management.

6. **Glial Cell Modulation**: Some research suggests that CBD may reduce the activation of glial cells in the spinal

cord and brain. Overactive glial cells have been implicated in chronic pain conditions.

It's important to note that while these mechanisms have been observed in laboratory and animal studies, more research is needed to fully understand how they translate to human pain experiences. Nonetheless, the multifaceted approach through which CBD appears to modulate pain makes it a promising area for further investigation in pain management.

Molecular Mechanisms of CBD's Anti-Inflammatory Effects

Inflammation is a key component of many pain conditions, and CBD's anti-inflammatory properties are a significant part of its therapeutic potential. Let's explore the molecular mechanisms behind these effects:

1. Inhibition of Pro-Inflammatory Cytokines

Cytokines are signaling proteins that play a crucial role in the inflammatory response. CBD has been shown to inhibit the production and release of pro-inflammatory cytokines, including:

- Tumor Necrosis Factor-α (TNF-α)

- Interleukin-1β (IL-1β)

- Interleukin-6 (IL-6)

By reducing the levels of these cytokines, CBD can help dampen the inflammatory response. This effect has been observed in various studies, including models of arthritis, inflammatory bowel disease, and multiple sclerosis.

2. Modulation of Immune Cell Function

CBD can influence the behavior of various immune cells involved in inflammation:

a) **T-cells**: CBD has been shown to suppress T-cell proliferation and reduce the production of pro-inflammatory cytokines by these cells.

b) **Macrophages**: CBD can modulate macrophage function, potentially shifting them from a pro-inflammatory state (M1) to an anti-inflammatory state (M2).

c) **Microglial Cells**: In the central nervous system, CBD can reduce the activation of microglial cells, which are involved in neuroinflammation.

3. NF-κB Pathway Inhibition

Nuclear factor kappa B (NF-κB) is a key transcription factor involved in inflammation. CBD has been shown to inhibit the NF-κB pathway, which in turn reduces the expression of pro-inflammatory genes.

4. Adenosine Enhancement

As mentioned earlier, CBD can enhance adenosine signaling. Adenosine has anti-inflammatory effects, and by increasing its levels, CBD may contribute to reducing inflammation.

5. PPARγ Activation

CBD's activation of PPARγ receptors can lead to the suppression of pro-inflammatory genes and the promotion of anti-inflammatory effects. This mechanism is particularly interesting because PPARγ agonists have shown promise in treating inflammatory conditions like inflammatory bowel disease.

6. Antioxidant Effects

While not directly an anti-inflammatory mechanism, CBD's antioxidant properties can contribute to reducing inflammation. Oxidative stress often accompanies and exacerbates inflammation, and by reducing oxidative damage, CBD may help mitigate the inflammatory response.

7. Modulation of Arachidonic Acid Pathways

Some studies suggest that CBD might influence the metabolism of arachidonic acid, a key player in the inflammatory process. By potentially reducing the production of pro-inflammatory eicosanoids, CBD could help dampen inflammation.

8. Endocannabinoid System Modulation

While CBD doesn't directly activate cannabinoid receptors, its ability to increase endocannabinoid levels (particularly anandamide) may contribute to its anti-inflammatory effects. The endocannabinoid system plays a role in regulating inflammation, and enhanced signaling in this system could help reduce inflammatory responses.

The Synergy of CBD's Actions

It's important to recognize that CBD's effects on pain and inflammation are not the result of a single mechanism, but rather the synergistic action of multiple pathways. This multi-target approach is part of what makes CBD so intriguing as a potential therapeutic agent.

For example, CBD's ability to reduce inflammation may indirectly contribute to pain relief by addressing one of the root causes of pain. Simultaneously, its direct effects on pain perception through modulation of receptors like TRPV1 and enhancement of endocannabinoid signaling provide additional paths for pain relief.

Moreover, CBD's anxiolytic effects could help break the cycle of pain and anxiety that often accompanies chronic pain conditions. By addressing both the physical and psychological aspects of pain, CBD offers a holistic approach to pain management.

While the mechanisms described in this chapter are backed by scientific research, it's crucial to note that much of this work has been done in laboratory and animal studies. Translating these findings to human clinical applications is an ongoing process.

Some challenges in understanding CBD's mechanisms include:

1. **Dose-Dependency**: CBD's effects can be biphasic, meaning different doses can produce different or even opposite effects. Understanding the optimal dosage for various conditions is an area of active research.

2. **Individual Variability**: Factors like genetics, overall health status, and the specific condition being treated can all influence how an individual responds to CBD.

3. **Entourage Effect**: Many researchers believe that CBD works best in conjunction with other cannabinoids and terpenes found in the cannabis plant. Understanding these

synergistic effects adds another layer of complexity to CBD research.

4. **Long-Term Effects**: More research is needed to fully understand the long-term effects of CBD use, both in terms of efficacy and potential side effects.

Despite these challenges, the multifaceted mechanisms of CBD's action offer exciting possibilities for pain and inflammation management. As research progresses, we may see more targeted applications of CBD based on its specific mechanisms of action.

Chapter 4

CBD for Common Pain Conditions

As we've explored in previous chapters, CBD's complex mechanisms of action offer potential benefits for various pain conditions. In this chapter, we'll look into four common pain conditions - arthritis, neuropathy, fibromyalgia, and migraines - and examine how CBD might play a role in their management. We'll look at the challenges each condition presents, review relevant research on CBD's efficacy, and include insights from both patients and experts in the field.

Arthritis

Description and Challenges:

Arthritis is not a single disease, but an umbrella term for joint pain or joint disease. The two most common types are osteoarthritis (OA) and rheumatoid arthritis (RA). Osteoarthritis is a degenerative condition where the cartilage that cushions the ends of bones wears away, leading to pain, stiffness, and swelling. Rheumatoid arthritis, on the other hand, is an autoimmune condition where the body's immune system attacks the joints, causing inflammation, pain, and potential joint deformity.

Challenges of arthritis include:

1. Chronic pain that can significantly impact quality of life

2. Reduced mobility and physical function

3. Difficulty performing daily activities

4. Side effects from long-term use of conventional treatments (e.g., NSAIDs, corticosteroids)

5. Progressive nature of the disease, particularly in RA

Research on CBD's Efficacy:

Several studies have investigated the potential of CBD in managing arthritis symptoms:

1. A 2016 study published in the European Journal of Pain used an animal model of arthritis to study the effects of transdermal CBD. The researchers found that CBD gel applied to the skin significantly reduced joint swelling and pain without evident side effects.

2. A 2017 study in the journal Pain examined CBD's effects on osteoarthritis pain in rats. The study found that CBD prevented the development of pain and nerve damage in osteoarthritic joints.

3. A 2018 review in Current Opinion in Pharmacology discussed the anti-inflammatory properties of cannabinoids, including CBD, and their potential in treating inflammatory diseases like arthritis.

4. A 2020 randomized controlled trial published in Pain Therapy looked at synthetic CBD in patients with hand osteoarthritis and psoriatic arthritis. While the results were mixed, some patients reported improvements in pain and function.

Patient Testimonial:

Joyce, 58, living with rheumatoid arthritis: "I've been dealing with RA for over a decade, and the pain has been debilitating at times. My rheumatologist suggested I try CBD oil as a complement to my current treatment. After about a month of consistent use, I noticed a significant reduction in my joint pain and stiffness, especially in the mornings. It's not a cure, but it's made a real difference in my day-to-day life."

Expert Opinion:

Dr. Jason McDougall, Professor of Pharmacology and Anesthesia at Dalhousie University: "There's certainly some promise there. The animal data is quite compelling, and we're starting to see some clinical evidence in humans as well. CBD's anti-inflammatory properties could be particularly beneficial for conditions like rheumatoid arthritis. However, we need more large-scale, well-designed clinical trials to fully understand its potential in arthritis management."

Neuropathy

Description and Challenges:

Neuropathy, or peripheral neuropathy, refers to damage or dysfunction of one or more nerves that typically results in numbness, tingling, muscle weakness, and pain in the affected area. It can result from various conditions, including diabetes, chemotherapy, injuries, infections, and certain medications.

Challenges of neuropathy include:

1. Chronic, often debilitating pain

2. Loss of sensation, which can lead to injuries

3. Muscle weakness and atrophy

4. Difficulty with balance and coordination

5. Resistance to many conventional pain medications

Research on CBD's Efficacy:

Several studies have explored CBD's potential in managing neuropathic pain:

1. A 2020 study published in Current Pharmaceutical Biotechnology reviewed the effects of cannabinoids on neuropathic pain. The authors concluded that CBD showed promise in treating neuropathic pain, both alone and in combination with other cannabinoids.

2. A 2017 study in Pain examined the effects of CBD in a rat model of neuropathic pain. The researchers found that

CBD treatment reduced pain and decreased anxiety-like behavior without causing analgesic tolerance.

3. A 2018 review in the British Journal of Pharmacology discussed the potential of cannabinoids, including CBD, in treating neuropathic pain. The authors noted that while more clinical trials are needed, preclinical evidence strongly supports the use of cannabinoids for neuropathic pain.

4. A small 2020 study published in Current Pharmaceutical Biotechnology looked at topical CBD oil in patients with peripheral neuropathy of the lower extremities. The study found a significant reduction in intense pain and sharp pain, as well as improvements in cold and itchy sensations.

Patient Testimonial:

Michael, 45, experiencing neuropathy due to chemotherapy: "The tingling and burning in my hands and feet were constant after my cancer treatment. Traditional pain meds helped a bit, but the side effects were rough. I started using CBD oil about six months ago, and it's been a game-changer. The pain is much more manageable now, and I've even been able to reduce my other pain medications. It's given me hope that I can get back to a more normal life."

Expert Opinion:

Dr. Ethan Russo, neurologist and cannabis researcher: "CBD has shown significant promise in treating neuropathic pain, which is often resistant to other treatments. Its ability to interact with multiple receptor systems involved in pain signaling makes it a particularly interesting candidate. While we need more clinical data, the preclinical evidence and early clinical studies are encouraging. CBD's favorable safety profile also makes it an attractive option for many patients."

Fibromyalgia

Description and Challenges:

Fibromyalgia is a chronic condition characterized by widespread musculoskeletal pain accompanied by fatigue, sleep, memory, and mood issues. The exact cause is unknown, but it's believed to involve how the brain and spinal cord process pain signals.

Challenges of fibromyalgia include:

1. Widespread, chronic pain

2. Fatigue and sleep disturbances

3. Cognitive difficulties (often called "fibro fog")

4. Mood disorders, including anxiety and depression

5. Comorbidity with other pain conditions

6. Lack of universally effective treatments

Research on CBD's Efficacy:

While research specifically on CBD for fibromyalgia is limited, there have been some promising studies:

1. A 2019 study published in Pain Medicine examined the effects of cannabis, which contains both CBD and THC, on fibromyalgia. The study found that cannabis use improved pain and other symptoms in some patients with fibromyalgia.

2. A 2020 review in Expert Opinion on Pharmacotherapy discussed the potential of cannabinoids in fibromyalgia management. The authors noted that while evidence is still limited, CBD's effects on pain and sleep could be beneficial for fibromyalgia patients.

3. A 2021 study in Clinical and Experimental Rheumatology looked at medical cannabis use in fibromyalgia patients. While this study wasn't specific to CBD, it found that cannabis use was associated with improvements in pain, sleep, and quality of life.

4. A 2018 review in the Journal of Clinical Medicine discussed the role of the endocannabinoid system in fibromyalgia and the potential of cannabinoids, including CBD, as a treatment option.

Patient Testimonial:

Emma, 37, living with fibromyalgia: "Fibromyalgia has been a daily struggle for years. The pain, fatigue, and brain fog made it hard to function. I started using CBD oil about a year ago, and while it's not a miracle cure, it's made a noticeable difference. My pain levels are lower, I'm sleeping better, and I feel more clear-headed during the day. It's helped me get back to doing things I love."

Description and Challenges:

Migraines are severe, recurring headaches often accompanied by other symptoms such as nausea, vomiting, sensitivity to light and sound, and visual disturbances. They can last for hours to days and significantly impact quality of life.

Challenges of migraines include:

1. Severe, debilitating pain

2. Unpredictability of attacks

3. Associated symptoms that can be as disruptive as the pain

4. Difficulty finding effective preventive treatments

5. Potential for medication overuse headaches with conventional treatments

Research on CBD's Efficacy:

Research on CBD specifically for migraines is still in its early stages, but some studies have shown promise:

1. A 2017 study presented at the 3rd Congress of the European Academy of Neurology looked at the use of cannabinoids for migraine prevention. While this study used a combination of THC and CBD, it found that cannabinoids were as effective as standard migraine preventive medications.

2. A 2019 review in Current Opinion in Neurology discussed the potential of cannabinoids in migraine treatment. The authors noted that while more research is needed, cannabinoids, including CBD, show promise for both acute and preventive migraine treatment.

3. A 2020 survey study published in Brain Sciences examined the use of cannabis, which often contains CBD, among migraine patients. Many participants reported that cannabis decreased the impact of migraines on their daily life.

4. A 2021 review in Neurotherapeutics discussed the role of the endocannabinoid system in migraine and the potential of cannabinoids, including CBD, as a treatment option.

Patient Testimonial:

Alex, 29, chronic migraine sufferer: "I've had migraines since I was a teenager, and they've always been hard to manage. I started using CBD oil daily about six months ago, and I've noticed a decrease in both the frequency and severity of my migraines. On days when I do get a migraine, using CBD alongside my usual medication seems to help it resolve faster. It's not a complete solution, but it's definitely improved my quality of life."

Chapter 5

Beyond Pain - CBD's Other Health Benefits

While CBD has garnered significant attention for its potential in pain management, its therapeutic reach extends far beyond analgesia. In this chapter, we'll explore three additional areas where CBD shows promise: anxiety and depression, sleep disorders, and skin health. These conditions not only impact overall well-being but often intersect with chronic pain, creating a complex web of symptoms that can significantly affect quality of life. We'll look into the research behind CBD's effects in these areas, examine potential mechanisms of action, and offer practical advice for those considering CBD for these purposes.

Anxiety and Depression

Connection to Pain and Overall Well-being:

Anxiety and depression often go hand in hand with chronic pain, creating a vicious cycle that can be challenging to break. Chronic pain can lead to anxiety and depression as individuals struggle with persistent discomfort and limitations in daily activities. Conversely, anxiety and depression can exacerbate pain perception, lower pain thresholds, and interfere with pain management strategies. This bidirectional relationship means that addressing mental health concerns can be crucial in managing chronic pain effectively.

Research Findings and Potential Mechanisms:

1. **Anxiety**:

Several studies have investigated CBD's anxiolytic (anti-anxiety) effects:

- A 2019 study published in the Journal of Clinical Medicine examined the effects of CBD on anxiety and sleep. The study found that CBD reduced anxiety scores in 79.2% of patients within the first month.

- A 2015 review in Neurotherapeutics analyzed CBD as a potential treatment for anxiety disorders. The authors concluded that preclinical evidence strongly supports CBD as a treatment for generalized anxiety disorder, panic disorder, social anxiety disorder, obsessive-compulsive disorder, and post-traumatic stress disorder.

- A 2011 study in the Journal of Psychopharmacology looked at CBD's effects on social anxiety disorder. Participants who received CBD before a public speaking test experienced significantly reduced anxiety, cognitive impairment, and discomfort compared to the placebo group.

Potential mechanisms for CBD's anxiolytic effects include:

- Interaction with serotonin 5-HT1A receptors, which are involved in anxiety and mood regulation.

- Modulation of GABA activity, enhancing the calming effects of this neurotransmitter.

- Promotion of neurogenesis in the hippocampus, which may help regulate mood and anxiety.

2. **Depression**:

While research on CBD for depression is still in early stages, some studies show promise:

- A 2018 study in Molecular Neurobiology found that CBD induced rapid and sustained antidepressant-like effects in animal models.

- A 2020 review in CNS & Neurological Disorders - Drug Targets discussed the potential of CBD in mood disorders, noting its antidepressant-like effects in preclinical studies.

- A 2019 study in the Journal of Chemical Neuroanatomy examined CBD's effects on depression and psychosis in animal models, finding that CBD exhibited antidepressant-like effects.

Potential mechanisms for CBD's antidepressant effects include:

- Enhancement of serotonin and glutamate signaling in the brain.

- Promotion of neuroplasticity and neurogenesis.

- Anti-inflammatory effects, as inflammation has been linked to depression.

Practical Advice for Using CBD for Anxiety and Depression:

1. Start Low and Go Slow: Begin with a low dose (e.g., 5-10mg) and gradually increase until you find the right balance of effects and side effects.

2. Consider the Delivery Method: For anxiety, sublingual oils or vaporized CBD may provide faster relief. For depression, daily supplementation with oils or capsules might be more suitable.

3. Be Consistent: Regular use may be more beneficial than sporadic use, especially for depression.

4. Timing Matters: For anxiety, taking CBD about an hour before stressful events might help. For depression, a consistent daily dose may be more effective.

5. Combine with Other Strategies: Use CBD as part of a comprehensive approach that includes therapy, exercise, and stress-reduction techniques.

6. Monitor Your Response: Keep a journal to track your symptoms, CBD dosage, and any changes you notice.

7. Consult a Professional: Always discuss CBD use with a healthcare provider, especially if you're taking other medications.

Sleep Disorders

Connection to Pain and Overall Well-being:

The relationship between sleep and pain is bidirectional and complex. Chronic pain can significantly disrupt sleep, leading to insomnia or poor sleep quality. Conversely, lack of sleep can lower pain thresholds and increase pain sensitivity. This creates a cycle where pain disturbs sleep, and poor sleep exacerbates pain. Moreover, sleep is crucial for overall health and well-being, affecting everything from cognitive function to immune health.

Research Findings and Potential Mechanisms:

Several studies have explored CBD's potential effects on sleep:

- The 2019 study in the Journal of Clinical Medicine mentioned earlier also looked at sleep scores. 66.7% of patients reported improved sleep within the first month of CBD use.

- A 2017 review in Current Psychiatry Reports discussed the potential of cannabinoids in treating sleep disorders. The authors noted that CBD might help with REM sleep behavior disorder and excessive daytime sleepiness.

- A 2014 study in Journal of Clinical Pharmacy and Therapeutics found that CBD could improve sleep in patients with Parkinson's disease.

- A 2016 case report in The Permanente Journal described a young girl with post-traumatic stress disorder and poor sleep who experienced a steady improvement in sleep quality with CBD oil.

Potential mechanisms for CBD's effects on sleep include:

- Reduction of anxiety, which can improve sleep onset and quality.

- Interaction with the endocannabinoid system, which plays a role in regulating sleep-wake cycles.

- Modulation of the release of sleep-related neurotransmitters.

Interestingly, CBD's effects on sleep might be biphasic, meaning low doses could be stimulating while higher doses are sedating.

Practical Advice for Using CBD for Sleep:

1. Timing is Key: Take CBD about an hour before bedtime to allow it to take effect.

2. Experiment with Dosage: Start low (e.g., 10-20mg) and increase gradually. Higher doses may be more effective for sleep.

3. Consider Full-Spectrum Products: The entourage effect from other cannabinoids and terpenes might enhance sleep benefits.

4. Be Consistent: Regular use may be more effective than occasional use for sleep improvement.

5. Combine with Sleep Hygiene: Use CBD as part of a comprehensive sleep routine that includes consistent sleep schedules, a dark and cool bedroom, and avoiding screens before bed.

6. Be Patient: It may take several weeks of consistent use to see significant improvements in sleep patterns.

7. Monitor Other Medications: CBD can interact with some sleep medications, so always consult with a healthcare provider.

Connection to Pain and Overall Well-being:

While skin health might seem disconnected from pain and overall well-being, it's more closely related than one might think. Skin conditions like acne, psoriasis, and eczema can cause significant discomfort and pain. Moreover, these conditions can impact self-esteem and quality of life, potentially contributing to stress, anxiety, and even depression. The skin is also our first line of defense against environmental stressors, playing a crucial role in overall health.

Research Findings and Potential Mechanisms:

CBD has shown promise in various aspects of skin health:

1. **Acne**:

- A 2014 study in the Journal of Clinical Investigation found that CBD exerted sebostatic and anti-inflammatory effects on human sebocytes, suggesting it could be a promising therapeutic agent for the treatment of acne vulgaris.

- A 2016 review in Experimental Dermatology discussed the potential of cannabinoids in skin disorders, noting CBD's anti-inflammatory and sebum-reducing properties.

2. Psoriasis:

- A 2019 study in La Clinica Terapeutica found that a CBD-enriched ointment improved skin parameters and symptoms in patients with psoriasis.

3. Eczema:

- While specific studies on CBD for eczema are limited, its anti-inflammatory properties suggest potential benefits.

4. Anti-Aging:

- A 2017 study in the Journal of the American Academy of Dermatology highlighted CBD's antioxidant properties, which could help combat signs of skin aging.

Potential mechanisms for CBD's effects on skin health include:

- Anti-inflammatory effects, reducing redness and swelling.

- Regulation of sebum production, potentially helping with acne.

- Antioxidant properties, combating free radical damage.

- Modulation of the endocannabinoid system in the skin, which plays a role in various skin processes.

Practical Advice for Using CBD for Skin Health:

1. Choose the Right Product: For skin health, topical CBD products like creams, lotions, or balms are often most effective.

2. Patch Test First: Always test a small amount on a small area of skin before applying more widely to check for any adverse reactions.

3. Be Consistent: Regular application is typically more effective than sporadic use.

4. Look for Additional Beneficial Ingredients: Many CBD skincare products also contain other skin-nourishing ingredients like hyaluronic acid or vitamins.

5. Consider Internal Use Too: While topical application can be beneficial, oral CBD might also support skin health from the inside out.

6. Be Patient: Skin changes can take time. Give the product at least a few weeks of consistent use before evaluating its effectiveness.

7. Combine with a Healthy Lifestyle: CBD can be part of a comprehensive skincare routine that includes a balanced diet, adequate hydration, and sun protection.

As we've explored in this chapter, CBD's potential benefits extend far beyond pain management. Its effects on anxiety, depression, sleep, and skin health highlight the compound's versatility and its potential to address multiple aspects of health and well-being simultaneously.

The interconnected nature of these health areas underscores the importance of a holistic approach to wellness. Anxiety and depression can exacerbate pain and sleep issues, poor sleep can worsen pain and mood disorders, and skin problems can impact self-esteem and overall quality of life. By potentially addressing multiple concerns, CBD offers an intriguing option for those seeking a more comprehensive approach to their health.

However, it's crucial to remember that while the research on CBD is promising, it's still in its early stages for many of these applications. Individual responses to CBD can vary, and what works for one person may not work for another. Moreover, CBD is not a replacement for professional medical care or a healthy lifestyle.

As with any supplement or medication, it's essential to approach CBD use thoughtfully and under the guidance of a healthcare provider. Factors like dosage, method of administration, and potential interactions with other medications all need to be considered. It's also important to source CBD products from reputable manufacturers who provide third-party lab testing results to ensure quality and purity.

Chapter 6

Integrating CBD into Your Pain Management Plan

As we've explored in previous chapters, CBD shows promising potential for pain management and overall wellness. However, incorporating CBD into your pain management routine requires careful consideration and planning. This chapter will guide you through the process of integrating CBD effectively, including how to determine the right dosage, choose the most suitable product type, and combine CBD with other natural pain relief strategies for a comprehensive approach to pain management.

Step-by-Step Guide for Determining Optimal CBD Dosage

One of the most challenging aspects of using CBD is determining the right dosage. Unlike many prescription medications, there's no standard, one-size-fits-all dose for CBD. The optimal amount can vary widely based on factors such as body weight, individual body chemistry, the condition being treated, and the concentration of CBD in the product you're using.

Here's a step-by-step guide to help you find your optimal CBD dosage:

Step 1: Start Low and Go Slow

The golden rule of CBD dosing is to start with a low dose and gradually increase it. This approach, often referred to as "titration," allows you to find the minimum effective dose for your needs while minimizing the risk of side effects.

Begin with a low dose of 5-10mg of CBD, taken once or twice daily. Maintain this dosage for about a week, paying close attention to how you feel.

Step 2: Monitor and Record Your Response

Keep a journal to track your CBD use and its effects. Note the following:

- The dose you're taking

- Time of day you're taking CBD

- Your pain levels before and after taking CBD

- Any changes in sleep, mood, or other symptoms

- Any side effects you experience

This information will be invaluable as you adjust your dosage.

Step 3: Gradually Increase the Dose

If you're not experiencing the desired effects after a week, increase your dose by 5-10mg. Continue this process of increasing the dose weekly and monitoring your response until you find the dose that provides optimal relief.

Step 4: Find Your Sweet Spot

Once you find a dose that provides good relief, you've found your "sweet spot." This is your optimal dose. For many people, this falls in the range of 20-40mg per day, but it can be lower or significantly higher for others.

Step 5: Consider Biphasic Effects

Be aware that CBD can have biphasic effects, meaning that higher doses don't always lead to increased benefits. In some cases, you might find that a lower dose actually works better. If you notice diminishing returns as you increase your dose, try scaling back.

Step 6: Adjust for Factors That May Influence CBD Metabolism

Several factors can influence how your body processes CBD:

- Body weight: Generally, people with higher body weight may need higher doses.

- Metabolism: If you have a fast metabolism, you might need to take CBD more frequently.

- The severity of symptoms: More severe pain might require higher doses.

- Tolerance: Some people develop a tolerance to CBD over time and may need to adjust their dose.

Step 7: Consult with a Healthcare Professional

Ideally, work with a healthcare provider experienced in CBD use. They can provide personalized guidance based on your specific health conditions and any medications you're taking.

Remember, finding your optimal CBD dosage is a process that requires patience and careful observation. It may take several weeks to find the right dose for you.

Comparing Different CBD Product Types

CBD comes in various forms, each with its own set of pros and cons. Understanding these can help you choose the product that best fits your needs.

1. CBD Oils and Tinctures

Pros:

- High bioavailability when taken sublingually (under the tongue)

- Easy to adjust dosage

- Fast-acting (15-30 minutes when taken sublingually)

- Long shelf life

Cons:

- Some people dislike the taste

- Can be messy

- May not be convenient for use in public

Best for: Those who want flexibility in dosing and fast-acting effects.

2. **CBD Capsules and Softgels**

Pros:

- Convenient and discreet

- Precise dosage

- No taste

- Easy to incorporate into existing supplement routine

Cons:

- Lower bioavailability than oils taken sublingually

- Slower to take effect (usually 30-90 minutes)

- Less flexibility in dosing

Best for: Those who prefer convenience and don't need to adjust their dose frequently.

3. **CBD Edibles (Gummies, etc.)**

Pros:

- Tasty and enjoyable to consume

- Discreet

- Pre-measured doses

Cons:

- Lower bioavailability due to digestion

- Slower onset of effects (can take 1-2 hours)

- Often contain added sugars

- Harder to adjust dosage precisely

Best for: Those who dislike the taste of CBD oil and don't mind a slower onset of effects.

4. CBD Topicals (Creams, Balms, etc.)

Pros:

- Can be applied directly to areas of pain

- Don't enter the bloodstream, so no risk of drug interactions

- Can be combined with other beneficial ingredients

Cons:

- Effects are localized

- Can be less potent for systemic issues

- Harder to gauge dosage

Best for: Localized pain and skin conditions.

5. **CBD Vape Products**

Pros:

- Highest bioavailability

- Fastest-acting (effects can be felt within minutes)

- Easy to adjust dosage

Cons:

- Effects don't last as long as other methods

- Potential respiratory risks associated with vaping

- Not suitable for those with lung conditions

Best for: Those needing very fast relief and comfortable with vaping.

When choosing a CBD product, consider factors like your lifestyle, the speed of onset you need, how long you need the effects to last, and any personal preferences regarding consumption method.

Complementary Natural Pain Relief Strategies and Combining with CBD

While CBD can be a powerful tool for pain management, it's most effective when used as part of a comprehensive pain management strategy. Here are some complementary natural pain relief approaches and how they can be combined with CBD:

1. Exercise and Physical Activity

Regular exercise can help reduce pain by strengthening muscles, improving flexibility, and releasing endorphins, the body's natural painkillers.

How to combine with CBD: Take CBD about an hour before exercise to potentially reduce exercise-induced inflammation and aid in recovery. CBD's potential anxiolytic effects might also help you feel more comfortable engaging in physical activity.

2. Mindfulness and Meditation

These practices can help change your perception of pain and reduce stress, which often exacerbates pain.

How to combine with CBD: Use CBD before meditation to potentially enhance relaxation and focus. CBD's calming effects might make it easier to engage in mindfulness practices.

3. Acupuncture

This traditional Chinese medicine technique has shown promise for various types of pain.

How to combine with CBD: Consider taking CBD before acupuncture sessions to potentially enhance relaxation and receptivity to treatment. Always inform your acupuncturist about your CBD use.

4. Yoga

Yoga combines physical postures, breathing techniques, and meditation, offering a holistic approach to pain management.

How to combine with CBD: Similar to exercise, taking CBD before yoga might help reduce exercise-induced inflammation and enhance the relaxation aspects of the practice.

5. Heat and Cold Therapy

Applying heat can relax muscles and increase blood flow, while cold can reduce inflammation and numb pain.

How to combine with CBD: Use CBD topicals in conjunction with heat or cold therapy for potentially enhanced effects. Apply the CBD product first, then apply heat or cold.

6. Herbal Supplements

Certain herbs like turmeric, ginger, and devil's claw have shown potential for pain relief.

How to combine with CBD: CBD can be taken alongside most herbal supplements, but always check for potential interactions. The anti-inflammatory effects of CBD might complement those of herbs like turmeric.

7. Dietary Changes

An anti-inflammatory diet rich in omega-3 fatty acids, fruits, vegetables, and whole grains may help reduce pain and inflammation.

How to combine with CBD: Incorporate CBD oil into your diet by adding it to smoothies, salad dressings, or other foods. The combination of an anti-inflammatory diet and CBD might offer synergistic benefits.

8. Massage Therapy

Massage can help reduce muscle tension, improve circulation, and promote relaxation.

How to combine with CBD: Use CBD-infused massage oils or creams during massage sessions for potentially enhanced relaxation and pain relief.

9. Sleep Hygiene

Good sleep is crucial for pain management, as poor sleep can lower pain thresholds.

How to combine with CBD: Consider taking CBD as part of your bedtime routine. Its potential to improve sleep quality might enhance your overall pain management strategy.

10. Stress Management Techniques

Stress can exacerbate pain, so techniques like deep breathing, progressive muscle relaxation, or biofeedback can be helpful.

How to combine with CBD: Use CBD to potentially enhance the relaxation effects of these techniques. CBD's anxiolytic properties might make it easier to engage in stress management practices.

When integrating CBD and these complementary strategies, keep the following tips in mind:

1. Start Slowly: When adding any new element to your pain management plan, introduce it gradually and one at a time. This allows you to gauge the effects of each addition clearly.

2. Keep a Journal: Track your pain levels, sleep quality, mood, and any other relevant factors as you integrate new strategies. This can help you identify what's most effective for you.

3. Be Consistent: Many of these strategies, including CBD use, are most effective when practiced consistently over time.

4. Listen to Your Body: Pay attention to how you feel and adjust your approach accordingly. What works best can vary from person to person.

5. Inform Your Healthcare Providers: Always keep your healthcare team informed about all elements of your pain management strategy, including CBD use and other complementary approaches.

6. Be Patient: Finding the right combination of strategies for your pain management can take time. Be patient with the process and with yourself.

7. Consider Professional Guidance: Working with a pain specialist, integrative medicine practitioner, or CBD-knowledgeable healthcare provider can provide valuable personalized guidance.

Chapter 7

Navigating the CBD Marketplace

The CBD industry has experienced explosive growth in recent years, with products ranging from oils and tinctures to edibles and topicals flooding the market. This rapid expansion has left many consumers feeling overwhelmed and unsure about how to choose high-quality, safe, and effective CBD products. In this chapter, we'll explore key strategies for navigating the CBD marketplace, including how to evaluate product quality, understand product labels and lab reports, and stay informed about the evolving legal landscape.

Evaluating CBD Product Quality: A Comprehensive Checklist

When shopping for CBD products, it's crucial to be discerning and well-informed. Use the following checklist to assess the quality and reliability of CBD products:

1. Source of hemp:

   - Is the hemp organically grown?

   - Is it cultivated in the United States or another country with strict agricultural regulations?

   - Does the company provide information about their farming practices?

2. Extraction method:

   - Is CO2 extraction or another clean method used?

   - Are any harsh solvents or chemicals employed in the process?

3. Full-spectrum, broad-spectrum, or isolate:

   - Does the product contain a full range of cannabinoids and terpenes?

   - If it's an isolate, is it pure CBD?

4. Third-party lab testing:

   - Are comprehensive lab reports readily available?

   - Do the reports confirm the advertised CBD content?

- Are the reports from a reputable, independent laboratory?

5. Ingredients:

   - Are all ingredients clearly listed on the label?

   - Are there any unnecessary additives or fillers?

   - For edibles or topicals, are the additional ingredients of high quality?

6. Potency:

   - Is the CBD concentration clearly stated?

   - Does the potency match your needs and experience level?

7. Company reputation:

   - How long has the company been in business?

   - Are there customer reviews available from verified purchasers?

   - Does the company have a good standing with consumer protection organizations?

8. Price and value:

- How does the price compare to similar products on the market?

- Is the price justified by the quality and potency of the product?

9. Packaging and presentation:

- Is the product packaged securely to prevent contamination or degradation?

- Is all necessary information clearly displayed on the label?

10. Customer service:

- Is it easy to contact the company with questions or concerns?

- Do they offer a satisfaction guarantee or return policy?

Deciphering CBD product labels and lab reports is essential for making informed purchasing decisions. Here's a detailed breakdown of what to look for:

Product Labels:

1. CBD content: Look for the total amount of CBD per container and per serving.

2. Serving size: Understand how much of the product constitutes a single serving.

3. Other cannabinoids: Check if THC, CBG, CBN, or other cannabinoids are present and in what quantities.

4. Ingredient list: All ingredients should be clearly listed, including carrier oils, flavorings, or other additives.

5. Batch or lot number: This allows you to match the product to its corresponding lab report.

6. Expiration date: Ensure the product is fresh and will remain potent for a reasonable period.

7. Usage instructions: Look for clear guidelines on how to use the product safely and effectively.

8. QR code or link to lab reports: Many reputable companies provide easy access to their third-party lab results.

Lab Reports (Certificates of Analysis):

1. Cannabinoid profile: This section details the concentrations of various cannabinoids, including CBD and THC.

2. Terpene profile: For full-spectrum or broad-spectrum products, this shows the types and amounts of terpenes present.

3. Contaminant testing: Look for results of tests for heavy metals, pesticides, residual solvents, and microbial contaminants.

4. Batch number: Ensure this matches the number on your product's label.

5. Testing facility information: Verify that the lab is accredited and independent from the manufacturer.

6. Date of analysis: Check that the testing was performed recently and matches the product's production timeline.

7. Potency analysis: Confirm that the CBD content aligns with what's advertised on the product label.

Understanding these elements will help you make more informed decisions and ensure you're getting a safe, high-quality CBD product that meets your needs.

Current Legal Status of CBD and Staying Informed

The legal landscape surrounding CBD is complex and evolving. As of 2024, here's a summary of the current situation:

1. **Federal level**:

   - The 2018 Farm Bill legalized hemp-derived CBD containing less than 0.3% THC.

   - The FDA still prohibits adding CBD to food or marketing it as a dietary supplement.

   - The FDA has approved one CBD-based prescription drug, Epidiolex, for certain seizure disorders.

2. **State level**:

   - Laws vary widely between states, with some fully embracing CBD and others maintaining stricter regulations.

- Some states have their own hemp programs with specific requirements for cultivation, testing, and sales.

3. **International**:

- Regulations differ significantly between countries, ranging from full legalization to complete prohibition.

- Always research local laws when traveling with CBD products.

To stay informed about changes in CBD legislation:

1. Follow reputable industry news sources and organizations such as:

   - The National Hemp Association

   - U.S. Hemp Roundtable

   - Project CBD

2. Monitor FDA and USDA websites for updates on federal regulations.

3. Check your state's health department or cannabis regulation board for local updates.

4. Subscribe to newsletters from trusted CBD companies and advocacy groups.

5. Attend industry conferences or webinars to learn about emerging trends and regulatory changes.

6. Consult with legal professionals specializing in cannabis law for personalized advice.

Navigating the CBD marketplace requires diligence, research, and a willingness to stay informed. By using the checklist provided, understanding product labels and lab reports, and keeping abreast of legal developments, you can make confident, educated decisions about CBD products. Remember that the industry is still maturing, and regulations are likely to continue evolving. Stay curious, ask questions, and prioritize transparency from CBD companies to ensure you're getting safe, high-quality products that meet your needs.

Chapter 8: The Future of CBD in Pain Management

The potential of CBD in pain management continues to captivate researchers, healthcare professionals, and patients alike. As our understanding of the endocannabinoid system deepens and research methodologies advance, we stand on the cusp of exciting developments in CBD-based therapies.

Exciting Areas of Ongoing CBD Research

The landscape of CBD research is rapidly evolving, with several key areas showing particular promise for pain management:

1. Chronic Pain Conditions:

Researchers are investigating CBD's efficacy in managing various chronic pain conditions, including fibromyalgia, neuropathic pain, and osteoarthritis. Early studies suggest that CBD may help modulate pain perception and reduce inflammation associated with these conditions.

2. **Cancer-Related Pain**:

CBD is being studied as a potential adjunct therapy for cancer-related pain, particularly in cases where traditional pain medications prove inadequate or cause severe side effects. Some research indicates that CBD may enhance the analgesic effects of opioids, potentially allowing for lower opioid doses.

3. **Migraine and Headache Disorders**:

Preliminary studies show promise for CBD in reducing the frequency and severity of migraines and cluster headaches. Researchers are exploring optimal dosing strategies and delivery methods for these applications.

4. **Autoimmune and Inflammatory Disorders**:

CBD's anti-inflammatory properties are being investigated for conditions like rheumatoid arthritis and inflammatory bowel diseases. Scientists are examining how CBD interacts with the immune system to potentially reduce pain and inflammation in these disorders.

5. **Post-Surgical Pain Management**:

There's growing interest in using CBD as part of multimodal pain management strategies following surgery. Studies are underway to determine if CBD can reduce the need for opioid pain medications during post-operative recovery.

6. Synergistic Effects with Other Cannabinoids:

The entourage effect, where multiple cannabinoids work together synergistically, is a key area of research. Scientists are exploring how CBD interacts with other cannabinoids like THC, CBG, and CBN to enhance pain relief while minimizing adverse effects.

7. Novel Delivery Methods:

Researchers are developing and testing new ways to deliver CBD for pain management, including transdermal patches, intranasal sprays, and sustained-release formulations. These innovations aim to improve bioavailability and provide more targeted pain relief.

8. Mechanism of Action Studies:

Ongoing research seeks to elucidate the precise mechanisms by which CBD affects pain perception and inflammation at the cellular and molecular levels. This foundational work is crucial for developing more effective and targeted CBD-based therapies.

Exploring Cannabinoid Pharmacogenomics

Cannabinoid pharmacogenomics is an emerging field that examines how an individual's genetic makeup influences their response to cannabinoids like CBD. This personalized medicine approach holds immense potential for optimizing CBD therapies for pain management:

1. Genetic Variations in the Endocannabinoid System:

Researchers are identifying genetic polymorphisms in cannabinoid receptors (CB1 and CB2) and enzymes involved in endocannabinoid metabolism. These variations may explain why some individuals respond more favorably to CBD than others.

2. Metabolism and Absorption:

Genetic differences in liver enzymes responsible for metabolizing CBD can affect how quickly the compound is processed and eliminated from the body. Understanding these variations could help in determining optimal dosing strategies for individuals.

3. Drug Interactions:

Pharmacogenomic studies are investigating how genetic factors influence potential interactions between CBD and other medications, particularly those metabolized by the cytochrome P450 enzyme system.

4. Predictive Biomarkers:

Scientists are working to identify genetic biomarkers that could predict an individual's likelihood of responding positively to CBD for pain management. This could help healthcare providers make more informed decisions about incorporating CBD into treatment plans.

5. Tailored Formulations:

As our understanding of cannabinoid pharmacogenomics grows, it may become possible to develop personalized CBD formulations that are optimized based on an individual's genetic profile.

6. Long-term Effects:

Researchers are exploring how genetic factors might influence the long-term effects of CBD use, including potential changes in endocannabinoid system function over time.

Strategies for Advocating CBD Use with Healthcare Providers

As interest in CBD for pain management grows, it's crucial to have productive conversations with healthcare providers about incorporating CBD into treatment plans. Here are strategies for effectively advocating for CBD use:

1. Do Your Research:

Before discussing CBD with your healthcare provider, arm yourself with credible, scientific information about CBD and its potential benefits for your specific condition. Bring peer-reviewed studies or reputable review articles to support your points.

2. Be Honest and Transparent:

If you're already using CBD, be upfront about your usage, including dosage, frequency, and any perceived benefits or side effects. This information is crucial for your provider to make informed decisions about your care.

3. Ask About Their Knowledge and Experience:

Inquire about your provider's familiarity with CBD and whether they have experience recommending it to other patients. This can help gauge their openness to the topic and identify any knowledge gaps.

4. Discuss Potential Drug Interactions:

If you're taking other medications, express your concerns about potential interactions with CBD. Ask your provider to review your current medication list and discuss any possible risks.

5. Request a Trial Period:

Suggest a monitored trial period where you incorporate CBD into your pain management regimen under your provider's supervision. Propose keeping a detailed journal of your symptoms, CBD usage, and any changes you notice.

6. Address Quality and Safety Concerns:

Discuss the importance of using high-quality, third-party tested CBD products. Ask for recommendations on reputable sources or if they can provide guidance on selecting safe products.

7. Explore Integrative Approaches:

Frame the discussion around integrating CBD into a comprehensive pain management plan rather than as a replacement for conventional treatments. This approach may be more palatable to providers who are hesitant about CBD.

8. Seek a Second Opinion if Necessary:

If your primary healthcare provider is unwilling to consider CBD, consider seeking a second opinion from a provider who specializes in integrative medicine or has experience with medical cannabis.

9. Stay Informed About Legal and Regulatory Issues:

Be prepared to discuss the legal status of CBD in your area and any relevant regulations that might affect its use in medical settings.

10. Follow Up and Provide Feedback:

If you do start using CBD with your provider's knowledge, schedule follow-up appointments to discuss your progress. Provide detailed feedback on your experience, which can help inform future treatment decisions.

The future of CBD in pain management is bright, with ongoing research promising to unlock new therapeutic possibilities. As the field of cannabinoid pharmacogenomics advances, we move closer to personalized CBD treatments that maximize efficacy while minimizing side effects. By staying informed about these developments and effectively communicating with healthcare providers, patients can play an active role in shaping the future of CBD-based pain management strategies. As always, it's crucial to approach CBD use as part of a holistic health plan, under the guidance of knowledgeable healthcare professionals.